PRE DIABETIC COOKBOOK FOR BEGINNERS

A Healthy Eating Guide, Easy Recipes, and Diabetes Meal Planner for Newly Diagnosed

Shelley Webster

Table of contents

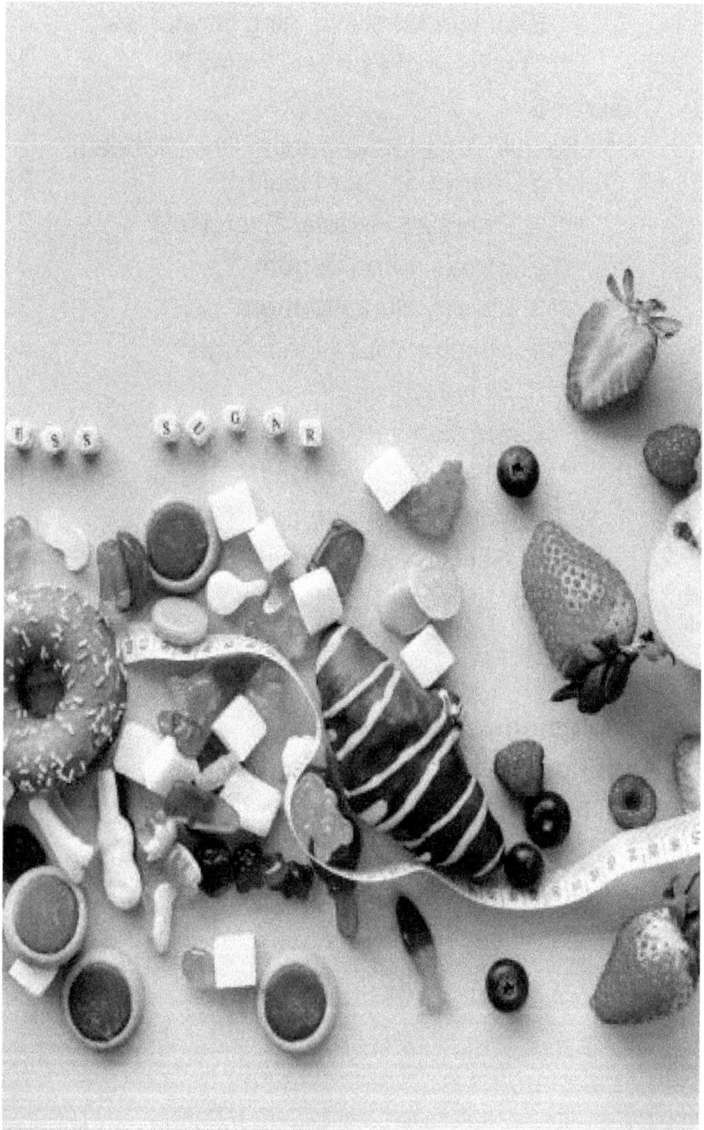
SUGAR

Introduction

Greetings from a revolutionary path to improved health and wellbeing.If you're holding this cookbook in your hands, it's likely that you, or someone you care about, has recently been diagnosed with pre-diabetes. We understand that this diagnosis can be a turning point in your life, but it's important to remember that it's also an opportunity for positive change.

Pre-diabetes is a condition that serves as a warning, a wake-up call that empowers you to take control of your health. The good news is that with the right knowledge and lifestyle choices, you can manage and even reverse pre-diabetes. And the cornerstone of this journey is your diet.

This cookbook is designed specifically for beginners like you, offering a wealth of information, delicious recipes, and practical guidance to help you navigate the world of pre-diabetes management. Here, we'll explore the foundations of a pre-diabetic diet, the importance of portion control, and the art of mindful eating. You'll find that eating healthfully doesn't have to mean compromising on flavor or pleasure.

Our recipes are tailored to not only manage your blood sugar but to tantalize your taste buds. You'll find a diverse array of dishes, from hearty breakfasts to satisfying dinners, with a selection of snacks and desserts that prove you don't have to give up the pleasures of eating.

But this cookbook isn't just about recipes. We'll also delve into the fundamentals of pre-diabetes, helping you understand the condition and its risk factors. You'll gain the confidence to make informed choices at the grocery store and while dining out. We'll discuss the vital role of exercise, stress management, and monitoring in your pre-diabetic journey.

Throughout this book, you'll find tools and resources to support your progress, from meal planning templates to quick-reference charts. The road to managing pre-diabetes may have started with a diagnosis, but it's your journey to better health that truly matters.

By taking this step toward a healthier, happier you, you're already on the path to success. We're here to be your companions on that journey, offering guidance and inspiration as you embrace a more balanced and vibrant life.

So, let's get started! Open the book, explore the pages, and embark on your pre-diabetic culinary adventure. Together, we'll prove that you can nourish your way to wellness and savor every step of the way.

Here's to your health, happiness, and a delicious future.

How to Take Control of Pre-Diabetes

The good news is that pre-diabetes is reversible and manageable through lifestyle changes. These key steps can help you regain control of your health:

1. ****Dietary Changes:**** Adopting a balanced, low-glycemic diet can help stabilize blood sugar levels. Focus on whole grains, lean proteins, and fiber-rich foods.

2. ****Physical Activity:**** Regular exercise is one of the most effective tools for managing pre-diabetes. Aim for at least 150 minutes of moderate aerobic activity each week.

3. ****Weight Management:**** Shedding excess weight, even a modest amount, can significantly improve your blood sugar control.

4. ****Stress Management:**** Chronic stress can elevate blood sugar levels. Practicing stress-reduction techniques like meditation and mindfulness can be beneficial.

5. ****Regular Monitoring:**** Keep track of your blood sugar levels, as recommended by your healthcare provider. Monitoring helps you assess the effectiveness of your lifestyle changes.

Understanding pre-diabetes is the first step toward a healthier, happier future. It's an opportunity to make informed choices about your health and well-being. With dedication and support, you can take charge of your pre-diabetic journey and reduce the risks of progression to full-blown diabetes. Remember, pre-diabetes is a warning, but it's also an invitation to take control of your health and embrace a brighter, more vibrant life.

The Importance of Diet and Lifestyle in Managing Pre-Diabetes

When it comes to managing pre-diabetes, two factors stand out as the cornerstones of success: diet and lifestyle. These elements are your most potent tools in the fight against this condition. Let's explore why they are crucial and how they can significantly impact your journey to better health.

Diet: The Foundation of Blood Sugar Control

Your diet plays a pivotal role in managing pre-diabetes. It directly influences your blood sugar levels, which, when unstable, can lead to the progression of this condition into type 2 diabetes. Here's why your dietary choices are so important:

1. **Blood Sugar Regulation:** The foods you consume have a direct impact on your blood sugar. Carbohydrates, in particular, can cause spikes if not managed correctly. A balanced diet can help keep blood sugar levels within a healthy range.

2. **Weight Management:** Maintaining a healthy weight is a key goal in managing pre-diabetes. Your diet affects your calorie intake, which, in turn, affects your weight. Healthy eating can help you

shed excess pounds and improve your insulin sensitivity.

3. **Nutrient Density:** A diet rich in essential nutrients such as vitamins, minerals, and fiber is crucial for overall health. It provides your body with the tools it needs to function optimally and combat the effects of pre-diabetes.

Lifestyle: The Engine of Positive Change

Your lifestyle choices go hand in hand with your dietary habits in managing pre-diabetes. These choices include physical activity, stress management, and more:

1. **Physical Activity:** Regular exercise is a potent weapon against pre-diabetes. It helps your body utilize glucose more efficiently, reduces insulin resistance, and supports weight management. Aim for a combination of aerobic and strength training exercises for the best results.

2. **Stress Management:** Chronic stress can elevate blood sugar levels. Learning to manage stress through techniques like meditation, yoga, or deep breathing can significantly improve your pre-diabetic condition.

3. **Sleep Hygiene:** A consistent sleep schedule and quality sleep are essential for blood sugar control. Poor sleep can lead to insulin resistance and weight gain, both of which are detrimental to managing pre-diabetes.

4. **Support and Accountability:** Your lifestyle choices are more sustainable when you have support from healthcare professionals, family, and friends. They can provide guidance, encouragement, and accountability on your journey.

By understanding the profound impact of diet and lifestyle, you can appreciate their significance in managing pre-diabetes. Your dietary choices can help regulate blood sugar and promote weight management, while lifestyle changes, including physical activity and stress reduction, can further enhance your journey toward better health.

Remember that managing pre-diabetes is not just about temporary changes. It's about adopting a sustainable, long-term approach to eating well and living healthily. With the right strategies and commitment, you can take control of your pre-diabetic condition and reduce the risk of progressing to full-blown diabetes. Your diet and lifestyle choices are your allies in this journey toward a brighter, healthier future

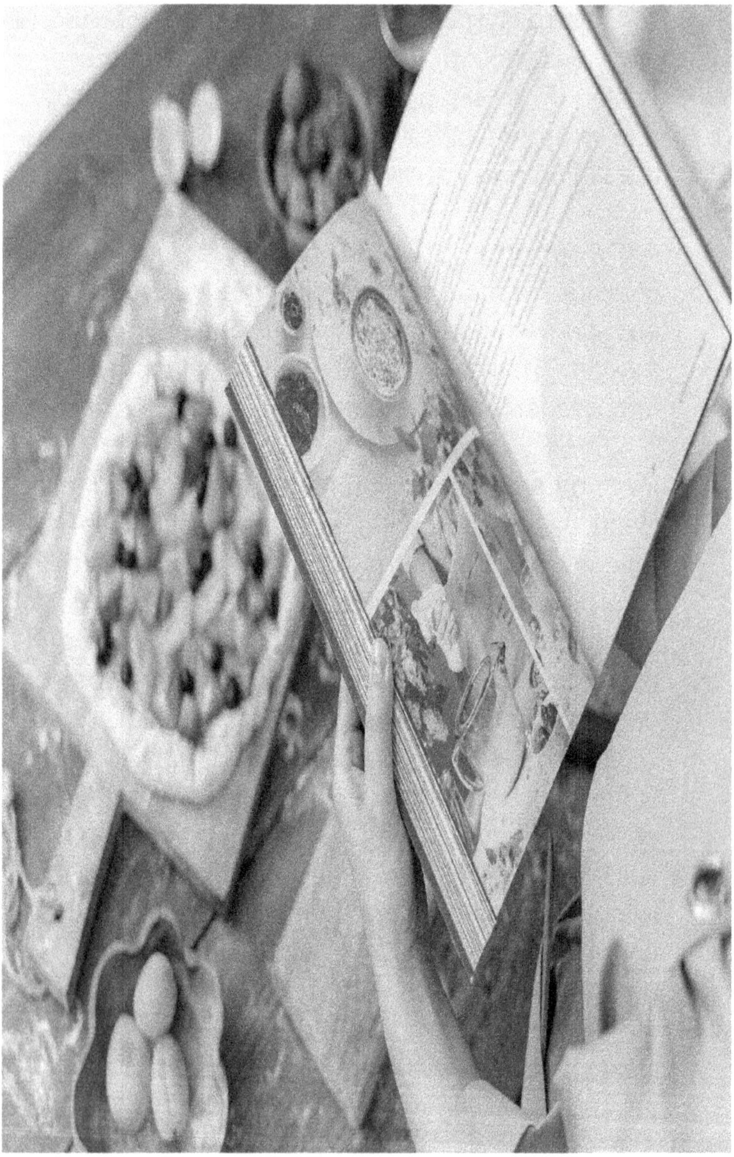

Chapter 1

Pre-Diabetes Explained: A Critical Stage in Your Health Journey

Pre-diabetes is a condition that often goes unnoticed, yet its implications for your health are profound. It serves as a warning, a call to action that should not be underestimated. To truly grasp what pre-diabetes means, it's important to understand the condition, its risk factors, and the significance of addressing it proactively.

What is Pre-Diabetes?

Pre-diabetes is a metabolic condition characterized by elevated blood sugar levels that are higher than normal but not yet in the range of diabetes. It's often referred to as a "gray area" where your body's ability to regulate blood sugar is compromised, but not to the extent of full-blown diabetes.
Pre-diabetes is typically diagnosed through a blood test, with one of the most common indicators being elevated HbA1c levels.

Why Does Pre-Diabetes Matter?

Pre-diabetes matters for several reasons:

1. **Progression to Diabetes:** Without intervention, many individuals with pre-diabetes eventually develop type 2 diabetes. This progression can lead to a range of health complications, including heart disease, stroke, kidney problems, and vision impairment.

2. **Silent Threat:** Pre-diabetes often goes unnoticed because it typically presents no symptoms. This means that you may feel perfectly healthy while the condition silently advances. Early detection is essential to preventing further complications.

3. **Risk Factors:** Multiple factors contribute to the development of pre-diabetes, including genetics, poor dietary choices, sedentary lifestyles, and obesity. Recognizing these risk factors can help you take preventive measures.

Understanding Risk Factors and Causes

Pre-diabetes doesn't occur in isolation. It's often the result of a combination of risk factors and causes, including:

1. **Weight:** Being overweight or obese is one of the primary risk factors for pre-diabetes. Excess fat, particularly around the abdomen, can contribute to insulin resistance.

2. **Physical Inactivity:** A sedentary lifestyle and lack of regular exercise can reduce your body's sensitivity to insulin, making it harder to control blood sugar.

3. **Dietary Choices:** A diet high in processed foods, sugary beverages, and refined carbohydrates can lead to blood sugar spikes and contribute to pre-diabetes.

4. **Genetics:** Family history can play a role. If you have close relatives with diabetes or pre-diabetes, your risk may be higher.

The Path To Reversal And Management

The good news is that pre-diabetes is often reversible through lifestyle changes. These changes include:

1. **Dietary Improvements:** A balanced diet that includes whole grains, lean proteins, fiber, and reduced sugar intake can help regulate blood sugar levels.

2. **Regular Exercise:** Incorporating physical activity into your routine, such as brisk walking or other forms of aerobic exercise, can significantly improve your insulin sensitivity.

3. **Weight Management:** Shedding excess weight, even a modest amount, can have a positive impact on your pre-diabetic condition.

4. **Monitoring:** Regular blood sugar monitoring, as recommended by your healthcare provider, is essential to track your progress.

Pre-diabetes is a condition that should not be taken lightly. It's a pivotal moment in your health journey, offering you the opportunity to make proactive choices that can positively impact your future. Understanding the condition, its risk factors, and the means of addressing it is the first step toward taking control of your health and preventing the progression to full-blown diabetes. With knowledge, determination, and support, you can navigate the path toward a healthier, happier life.

Chapter 2

Pre-Diabetic Diet Basics: Nourishing Your Way to Better Health

A pre-diabetes diagnosis is a wake-up call, urging you to make important changes to your lifestyle, especially your diet. Fortunately, understanding the fundamentals of a pre-diabetic diet can empower you to take control of your health and make choices that can prevent the progression to type 2 diabetes. Let's explore the essential elements of a pre-diabetic diet.

1. Balanced Plate Approach

The cornerstone of a pre-diabetic diet is achieving balance in your meals. Aim to create a plate that consists of:

- **Half Non-Starchy Vegetables:** Fill your plate with colorful vegetables like broccoli, spinach, bell peppers, and cauliflower. These are low in carbohydrates and rich in essential nutrients.

- **One-Quarter Lean Proteins:** Incorporate lean protein sources such as skinless poultry, fish, tofu, or legumes. Proteins help control your appetite and stabilize blood sugar.

- **One-Quarter Whole Grains or Starchy Vegetables:** Opt for whole grains like quinoa, brown rice, or sweet potatoes. These provide fiber and carbohydrates that are slower to digest, preventing blood sugar spikes.

2. Carbohydrates and Blood Sugar Control

Carbohydrates play a central role in blood sugar management for pre-diabetics. Pay attention to the type and quantity of carbs in your diet:

- **Choose Complex Carbs:** Prioritize complex carbohydrates found in whole grains, legumes, and vegetables over simple sugars. These are digested more slowly, preventing rapid blood sugar spikes.

- **Control Portion Sizes:** Be mindful of portion sizes when consuming carbohydrate-rich foods. Measuring portions and using smaller plates can help prevent overeating.

- **Fiber is Key:** **High**-fiber foods like oats, beans, and vegetables can help stabilize blood sugar. Aim for at least 25 grams of fiber per day.

3. Fiber-Rich Foods

Fiber is a pre-diabetic's best friend. It helps slow down the absorption of sugar in the bloodstream, preventing blood sugar spikes:

- **Soluble Fiber:** Found in foods like oats, apples, and legumes, soluble fiber forms a gel in the stomach, which slows digestion and reduces the impact on blood sugar.

- **Insoluble Fiber:** This type, present in whole grains and vegetables, adds bulk to your diet, promoting a feeling of fullness and preventing overeating.

4. Sugar and Processed Foods

Reducing added sugars and processed foods is crucial for pre-diabetic individuals:

- **Read Labels:** Check food labels for hidden sugars, such as high fructose corn syrup or other sugar derivatives. Aim for products with little to no added sugars.

- **Limit Processed Foods:** Highly processed foods often contain unhealthy fats, excessive sugars, and refined carbohydrates. Opt for whole, unprocessed options.

5. Healthy Fats

Healthy fats are an essential part of a balanced diet:

- ***Monounsaturated and Polyunsaturated** Fats:** Found in olive oil, avocados, and fatty fish like salmon, these fats can help reduce the risk of heart disease.

- **Limit Saturated and Trans Fats:** Reducing your intake of saturated and trans fats, typically found in fried foods and processed snacks, is important for heart health.

6. Meal Timing and Consistency

Maintaining regular meal times and avoiding long gaps between meals can help stabilize blood sugar levels. Aim for three balanced meals and healthy snacks if needed.

7. Hydration

Staying hydrated is key. Water helps your body process glucose efficiently and supports overall health. Make it a point to stay hydrated throughout the day.

Remember that a pre-diabetic diet is not about deprivation but rather about making informed choices that promote your health and well-being. It's a journey toward a more balanced and vibrant life. By understanding these diet basics and implementing them into your daily routine, you're taking a significant step toward managing pre-diabetes and preventing its progression to type 2 diabetes. With the right knowledge and commitment, you can nourish your way to a healthier future.

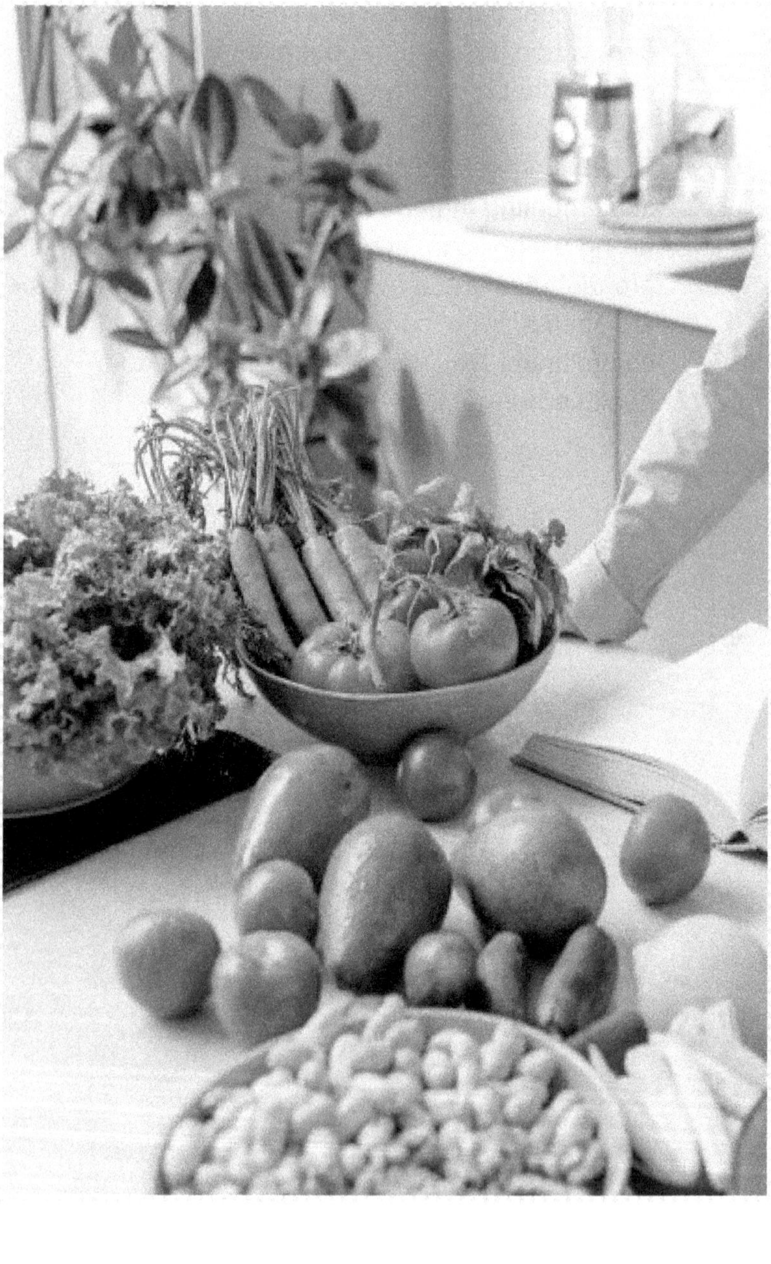

Chapter 3

Grocery Shopping for Success: A Pre-Diabetic's Guide to Healthy Eating

A trip to the grocery store can be a pivotal moment in your pre-diabetic journey. The choices you make here can significantly impact your health and well-being. To ensure success, it's essential to approach grocery shopping with a plan. Here's how to navigate the aisles for pre-diabetic-friendly foods.

1. Prepare a Shopping List

Before heading to the store, take a few minutes to create a shopping list. A list not only ensures you get everything you need but also helps you avoid impulse purchases that may not align with your pre-diabetic diet.

Include items like fresh vegetables, lean proteins, whole grains, and low-fat dairy if applicable. Be specific about the quantities you need to prevent over-purchasing.

2. Shop the Perimeter

As a general rule, focus on the outer aisles of the store. This is where you'll find fresh produce, lean meats, and dairy products. The perimeter is usually home to the most natural, unprocessed foods, making it the heart of a pre-diabetic-friendly diet.

3. Read Nutritional Labels

When you venture into the inner aisles of the store, where packaged and processed foods are found, be a discerning shopper. Read nutritional labels to identify products with excessive added sugars, unhealthy fats, and high carbohydrate content. Look for foods that are lower in added sugars and saturated fats.

4. Choose Whole Grains

Opt for whole grains like brown rice, quinoa, and whole wheat pasta. These grains are less processed, maintaining their fiber content and resulting in slow digestion and better blood sugar control.

5. Fresh Produce is King

Load your cart with fresh, colorful fruits and vegetables. These nutrient-packed foods are rich in fiber and essential vitamins and minerals. They should be the centerpiece of your pre-diabetic diet.

6. Lean Proteins

Select lean protein sources like skinless poultry, fish, lean cuts of beef or pork, and plant-based proteins like tofu and legumes. Protein helps stabilize blood sugar and keeps you feeling full.

7. Dairy or Dairy Alternatives

If you consume dairy, choose low-fat or fat-free options. Otherwise, opt for unsweetened dairy alternatives like almond or soy milk. Be cautious with flavored or sweetened versions, as they may contain added sugars.

8. Healthy Fats

Look for sources of healthy fats, such as avocados, nuts, seeds, and olive oil. These fats are good for your heart and overall health.

9. Cautious with Snacks

When selecting snacks, choose wisely. Nutrient-dense options like whole fruits, unsalted nuts, and Greek yogurt are preferable to processed snacks high in added sugars and unhealthy fats.

10. Avoid Sugary Drinks

Steer clear of sugary beverages like soda and fruit juices, as they can cause rapid blood sugar spikes. Opt for water, herbal tea, or unsweetened sparkling water.

11. Be Mindful of Portion Sizes

Even healthy foods can affect blood sugar if consumed in excessive quantities. Pay attention to portion sizes, and consider buying smaller plates to help with portion control at home.

12. Stock Up on Staples

Don't forget pantry staples like beans, lentils, and whole-grain pasta. These are versatile ingredients that can be used in a variety of pre-diabetic-friendly recipes.

By approaching grocery shopping with a plan and a keen eye for nutritious choices, you can set yourself up for success in managing pre-diabetes. These thoughtful selections not only help regulate your blood sugar but also contribute to your overall health and well-being. Over time, you'll develop a routine that aligns with your pre-diabetic diet, making healthy eating a sustainable part of your lifestyle.

Chapter 4

Pre-Diabetes Friendly Recipes: Delicious and Nutritious Choices for Better Health

Eating well with pre-diabetes doesn't mean giving up on flavorful and satisfying meals. In fact, it's an opportunity to explore a world of delicious, pre-diabetic-friendly recipes that support your health and well-being. Let's dive into the culinary journey of creating tasty dishes that keep your blood sugar in check.

1. Breakfast Delights

Starting your day with a balanced and satisfying breakfast is key to managing pre-diabetes. Here are a couple of recipes that provide a hearty morning boost:

- *Low-Glycemic Oatmeal*: Swap instant oats for steel-cut oats and top with fresh berries and a sprinkle of cinnamon for a filling and slow-release energy breakfast.

- *Avocado and Egg Breakfast*: Poach or scramble an egg and serve it over half an avocado with a sprinkle of black pepper. This protein-packed breakfast will keep you feeling full and energized.

2. Lunchtime Favorites

Lunch should be a balanced, midday refueling opportunity. Try these recipes:

- *Quinoa and Vegetable Salad*: Cook quinoa and toss it with a colorful mix of fresh vegetables, such as bell peppers, cucumbers, and cherry tomatoes. Drizzle with a light vinaigrette dressing.

- *Turkey and Avocado Wrap*: Use whole-grain wraps and fill them with lean turkey slices, sliced avocado, lettuce, and a touch of low-fat Greek yogurt.

3. Dinner Options

Dinner can be a satisfying, pre-diabetic-friendly affair. These recipes showcase flavorful, wholesome options:

- *Baked Salmon with Garlic Roasted Veggies*: Season salmon fillets with herbs and roasted alongside a medley of your favorite vegetables, such as broccoli, zucchini, and carrots. Drizzle with olive oil and sprinkle minced garlic.

- *Lentil and Vegetable Stew*: Simmer lentils, diced tomatoes, and a variety of vegetables like bell peppers, spinach, and onions in a flavorful broth.

Season with herbs and spices for a nutritious, fiber-rich stew.

4. Snacks and Side Dishes

Between meals, these recipes can serve as snacks or sides:

- ***Greek Yogurt with Berries*:** A bowl of plain Greek yogurt topped with fresh berries and a drizzle of honey is a satisfying and protein-rich snack.

- ***Roasted Chickpeas*:** Toss chickpeas with olive oil and your favorite spices, then roast until they're crispy for a crunchy and high-fiber snack.

5. Sweet Treats

Managing pre-diabetes doesn't mean giving up on sweet treats entirely. Try these healthier alternatives:

- ***Sugar-Free Fruit Popsicles*:** Blend your favorite fruits with water and a touch of stevia or another sugar substitute, then freeze in molds for a refreshing treat.

- ***Dark Chocolate-Dipped Strawberries*:** Melt dark chocolate (70% cocoa or higher) and dip fresh strawberries for a delicious yet lower-sugar dessert.

Each of these recipes emphasizes whole, unprocessed ingredients, high fiber content, lean proteins, and low-glycemic options. They are designed to support your blood sugar management while delighting your taste buds.

Remember, portion control remains important. Eating mindfully, paying attention to portion sizes, and spreading your meals throughout the day can help keep your blood sugar levels stable. Pre-diabetic-friendly recipes aren't just about what you eat but how you eat, too.

With these recipes and a commitment to your pre-diabetic journey, you can discover that healthy eating can be a flavorful and satisfying part of your lifestyle. Enjoy the journey to better health through delicious, pre-diabetic-friendly recipes!

Chapter 5

Meal Planning and Portion Control: The Key to Pre-Diabetes Management

When you're dealing with pre-diabetes, every meal becomes an opportunity to take control of your health. Meal planning and portion control are the guiding principles that ensure you make wise food choices and maintain stable blood sugar levels. Let's explore why these strategies are so important and how you can implement them effectively.

The Importance of Meal Planning

Meal planning is the proactive process of deciding what to eat, when to eat, and how much to eat in advance. It offers several vital benefits for pre-diabetic individuals:

1. **Balanced Nutrition:** Planning your meals allows you to ensure that each one is well-balanced with the right mix of carbohydrates, proteins, and fats.

2. ***Portion Control:*** You can determine appropriate portion sizes to prevent overeating and blood sugar spikes.

3. ****Blood Sugar Stability:**** By selecting low-glycemic foods and avoiding large fluctuations in your diet, meal planning can help stabilize blood sugar levels.

*4. ****Avoiding Impulsive Consumption:****
Having a plan in place reduces the chances of making unhealthy, impulsive food choices.

Effective Meal Planning Strategies

To get started with meal planning, consider these strategies:

1. ****Plan Ahead:**** Take time each week to plan your meals and snacks. Consider your schedule and activities to ensure you have appropriate food available.

*2. ****Include Variety:**** Incorporate a variety of foods to make your meals enjoyable and nutritionally balanced.

*3. ****Portion Control:**** Be mindful of portion sizes. Use measuring cups and kitchen scales if needed to avoid overeating.

*4. ****Smart Snacking:**** Plan for nutritious snacks in between meals to prevent excessive hunger and poor food choices.

5. **Mindful Grocery Shopping:** Create a shopping list based on your meal plan and stick to it. Avoid impulse buying.

The Role of Portion Control

Portion control is fundamental for pre-diabetic individuals. It helps you manage your caloric intake and prevents overeating, which can lead to blood sugar spikes. Here's how you can implement effective portion control:

1. **Use Smaller Plates:** Smaller plates and bowls can make portion sizes look more substantial, reducing the temptation to load your plate with excess food.

2. ***Divide Your Plate:*** Follow the balanced plate approach mentioned in a previous response. This strategy, which includes non-starchy vegetables, lean proteins, and whole grains or starchy vegetables, ensures portion control while promoting a balanced diet.

3. **Avoid Eating from Containers:** Instead of snacking directly from a bag of chips or a box of cookies, portion out a serving and put the container away to prevent mindless overeating.

4. ***Learn Portion Sizes:*** Educate yourself about standard portion sizes for different foods, and use

measuring tools until you become proficient at estimating portion sizes accurately.

*5. **Practice Mindful Eating*:** Pay attention to your food while you eat. Savor each bite and chew slowly, which can help you feel full with less food.

Effective meal planning and portion control empower you to make healthier choices, maintain stable blood sugar levels, and support your journey in managing pre-diabetes. With practice and commitment, these strategies will become second nature, leading you toward better health and well-being.

Chapter 6

Lifestyle Tips for Managing Pre-Diabetes: Taking Charge of Your Health

Pre-diabetes doesn't have to be a one-way path to type 2 diabetes. With the right lifestyle adjustments, you can take control of your health and reduce the risk of progression. Here are some lifestyle tips to help you effectively manage pre-diabetes:

1. Prioritize Regular Exercise

Physical activity is one of the most potent tools for managing pre-diabetes. Regular exercise offers several benefits:

- **Improved Insulin Sensitivity:** Physical activity helps your body use insulin more efficiently, which is crucial for blood sugar control.

- **Weight Management:** Exercise supports weight loss or maintenance, reducing a key risk factor for pre-diabetes.

- ***Stress Reduction:*** Physical activity can help manage stress, which plays a role in blood sugar regulation.

Aim for at least 150 minutes of moderate aerobic activity per week, along with strength training exercises.

2. Stress Management

Chronic stress can elevate blood sugar levels and contribute to pre-diabetes. Incorporate techniques for reducing stress into your daily activities:

- ***Mindfulness and Meditation:*** Practices like meditation, deep breathing, and mindfulness can help reduce stress levels.

- ***Yoga:*** Yoga combines physical activity with relaxation techniques, making it an excellent choice for stress reduction.

- ***Time Management:*** Organize your schedule to prioritize self-care and relaxation.

3. Quality Sleep Matters

Consistent, quality sleep is essential for managing pre-diabetes. Poor sleep can lead to insulin resistance, weight gain, and poor blood sugar control. Establish a sleep routine with a consistent bedtime and wake-up time.

4. Monitor Your Blood Sugar

Regular blood sugar monitoring is key to understanding how your choices impact your pre-diabetic condition. Your healthcare provider can guide you on when and how often to check your levels.

5. Stay Hydrated

Water plays a significant role in glucose processing. Staying well-hydrated can help your body process glucose more efficiently.

6. Supportive Communities

Joining a support group or participating in online communities can provide valuable encouragement and advice. Sharing your experiences and learning from others can be motivating and reassuring.

7. Regular Check-Ups

Schedule regular check-ups with your healthcare provider. They can monitor your progress, adjust your treatment plan if needed, and provide essential guidance.

8. Weight Management

Shedding excess weight, even a modest amount, can significantly improve your blood sugar control.

Focus on balanced, low-glycemic meals and regular exercise to help with weight management.

9. Set Realistic Goals

Set achievable goals for yourself. Whether it's adding an extra day of exercise or including more vegetables in your meals, small, realistic changes can lead to significant improvements over time.

10. Stay Informed

Continuously educate yourself about pre-diabetes. Knowledge is a powerful tool for making informed choices and staying motivated.

Remember, managing pre-diabetes is a journey, not a destination. By embracing these lifestyle tips and making gradual, sustainable changes, you can take control of your health, reduce the risks of developing type 2 diabetes, and enjoy a healthier, happier life. Each positive choice you make brings you one step closer to better well-being.

Chapter 7

Variety

In the world of managing pre-diabetes, variety isn't just the spice of life; it's a fundamental ingredient. Embracing a diverse range of foods and recipes not only makes your journey more enjoyable but also plays a pivotal role in maintaining steady blood sugar levels.

Variety in your diet serves multiple essential purposes when you're on the path to managing pre-diabetes. Let's explore why it's a cornerstone of success:

****Balanced Nutrition:**** Each food brings a unique set of nutrients to the table. By including a variety of foods, you're more likely to achieve a balanced intake of essential vitamins, minerals, fiber, and antioxidants.

****Flavor and Satisfaction:**** Relying on a narrow selection of foods can lead to boredom and cravings, making it harder to stick to your dietary plan. A varied diet keeps your taste buds engaged and satisfied.

****Blood Sugar Stability:**** Different foods have different effects on blood sugar levels. Incorporating a range of low-glycemic index foods helps stabilize glucose, preventing sharp spikes or drops.

Nutritional Resilience: Variety in your diet prepares you for life's twists and turns. Whether it's dining out, traveling, or dealing with food allergies, having a repertoire of pre-diabetic-friendly options gives you flexibility.

Preventing Nutrient Gaps: Each food offers a unique profile of nutrients. By including a variety, you reduce the risk of missing out on vital vitamins and minerals.

Avoiding Monotony: Eating the same foods daily can lead to burnout and decreased compliance with your dietary plan. Variety keeps your meals exciting and sustainable.

Here's how you can embrace variety in your pre-diabetic diet:

1. **Explore New Foods:** Don't be afraid to try ingredients you've never used before. There's a whole world of delicious, healthy options waiting for you.

2. **Seasonal Eating:** Take advantage of seasonal fruits and vegetables. They offer freshness and variety throughout the year.

3. **Colorful Plates:** Aim to fill your plate with a variety of colors. Different colors often signify different nutrient profiles.

4. **Cuisine Adventure:** Experiment with international cuisines. Each culture brings its unique flavors and ingredients to the table.

5. **Recipe Exploration:** try a wide range of recipes. From savory to sweet, there's a world of options to discover.

Remember, variety is your ally in this journey, not a challenge. It empowers you to make pre-diabetic-friendly choices while enjoying a diverse, flavorful, and nutritious diet. By embracing variety, you're not just managing pre-diabetes; you're savoring the delightful array of culinary possibilities that support your path to better health.

When choosing a pre-diabetic cookbook or resource, it's essential to consider your personal dietary preferences, any specific dietary restrictions you may have, and the level of guidance you're seeking. Additionally, consult with a healthcare provider or a registered dietitian to develop a personalized dietary plan that aligns with your unique needs. These pre-diabetic cookbook resources, combined with professional guidance, can be powerful tools in managing pre-diabetes through a delicious and balanced diet.

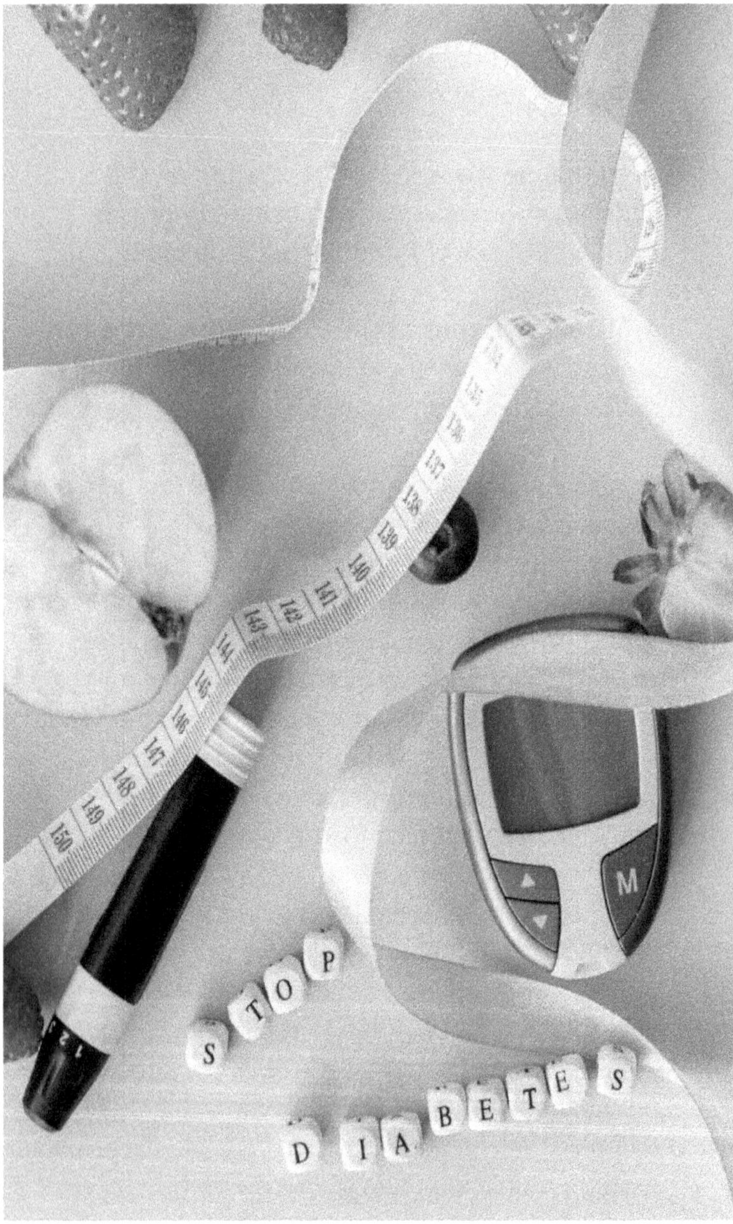
STOP
DIABETES

Conclusions

In conclusion, managing pre-diabetes is a crucial step in safeguarding your health and preventing the progression to type 2 diabetes. You do not have to embark on this trip by yourself. By understanding the condition, embracing a pre-diabetic-friendly diet, and adopting a healthier lifestyle, you can take control of your well-being.

Remember the key points:

1. **Pre-Diabetes Awareness:** Recognizing the condition's existence is the first step. Understanding what pre-diabetes is, its risk factors, and its implications is vital to your health journey.

2. **Diet and Lifestyle:** Diet and lifestyle choices are your most potent allies in managing pre-diabetes. A balanced diet, regular exercise, stress management, and quality sleep are your cornerstones for success.

3. **Portion Control:** Learning to control your portion sizes can help prevent overeating, stabilize blood sugar, and promote weight management.

4. **Meal Planning:** Strategically planning your meals and snacks empowers you to make

nutritious choices and maintain stable blood sugar levels.

5. **Lifestyle Tips:** Stay informed and embrace a supportive community. Regular check-ups with healthcare providers are essential for monitoring your progress.

With these strategies and the commitment to your well-being, you have the power to manage pre-diabetes effectively. By making informed choices and embracing a balanced, healthy lifestyle, you're taking a proactive step toward a healthier and happier future. Your journey is a testament to your strength, determination, and dedication to your health.

Appendix Quick References Guide

Glycemic Index Chart

Certainly! Here's a simplified Glycemic Index (GI) chart featuring various common foods. The GI indicates how quickly a food raises blood sugar levels. Low-GI foods are digested slowly, leading to gradual blood sugar increases, while high-GI foods cause rapid spikes. Remember that this chart is a general reference; individual responses to foods may vary.

Low-GI Foods (55 or less)
- Non-starchy vegetables (e.g., broccoli, spinach, kale)
- Legumes (e.g., lentils, chickpeas, black beans)
- Whole grains (e.g., quinoa, barley, whole wheat)
- Sweet potatoes
- Nuts and seeds
- Most fruits (e.g., apples, berries, cherries)
- Whole-grain pasta

Medium-GI Foods (56-69)
- Whole wheat bread
- Basmati rice
- Oatmeal
- Brown rice

- Pineapple
- Raisins
- Couscous

High-GI Foods (70 or more)
- White bread
- White rice
- Instant oatmeal
- Cornflakes
- Watermelon
- Sugary cereals
- Pretzels
- French fries

It's important to note that the glycemic index of a food can be influenced by factors like ripeness, cooking methods, and food combinations. For precise GI values, refer to reputable glycemic index databases and resources. When managing pre-diabetes, aim to prioritize low-GI and moderate-GI foods to help stabilize blood sugar levels.

Food Substitution List

Certainly! Here's a food substitution list to help you make healthier choices when managing pre-diabetes. Substituting high-GI or high-sugar foods with lower-GI alternatives can be beneficial for blood sugar control.

Instead of White Rice, Choose:

- Brown rice
- Quinoa
- Cauliflower rice

Instead of White Bread, Choose:
- Whole-grain bread
- Whole wheat pita
- Rye bread

Instead of Sugary Cereals, Choose:
- Oatmeal (plain, not instant)
- Whole-grain cereals with no added sugar
- Low-sugar muesli

Instead of Sugary Snacks, Choose:
- Fresh fruit
- Greek yogurt with berries
- Mixed nuts (in moderation)

Instead of Soda or Sugary Drinks, Choose:
- Water
- Herbal tea
- Sparkling water with a twist of lemon or lime

Instead of Potato Chips, Choose:
- Baked sweet potato chips
- Air-popped popcorn
- Veggie sticks with hummus

Instead of Ice Cream, Choose:
- Greek yogurt with honey and fresh fruit
- Frozen yogurt with no added sugar

- Sorbet

Instead of Candy, Choose:
- Dark chocolate (70% cocoa or higher)
- Fresh or dried fruit
- Nut butter on whole-grain crackers

Instead of Sugary Condiments, Choose:
- Olive oil and vinegar for salads
- Mustard instead of ketchup
- Low-sugar or no-sugar-added options

Instead of Full-Fat Dairy, Choose:
- Low-fat or fat-free dairy products
- Unsweetened dairy alternatives (almond, soy, or coconut milk)
- Greek yogurt (plain or low-fat)

Instead of Fried Foods, Choose:
- Baked or grilled options
- Oven-baked sweet potato fries
- Steamed or stir-fried dishes

Instead of High-Sugar Sauces, Choose:
- Tomato sauce with no added sugar
- Homemade pesto with less oil
- Low-sodium soy sauce

Instead of High-Sugar Breakfast Cereals, Choose:
- Unsweetened oatmeal
- Whole-grain bran flakes

- Plain shredded wheat

Remember, these substitutions can help you make healthier choices and manage pre-diabetes, but portion control is also essential. Additionally, individual dietary preferences and tolerances should be considered when making these substitutions. Always consult with a healthcare provider or a registered dietitian for personalized dietary advice.

Here's a simple weekly meal planner template that you can use to help organize your meals when managing pre-diabetes. You can print it out or use it digitally to plan your breakfast, lunch, dinner, and snacks:

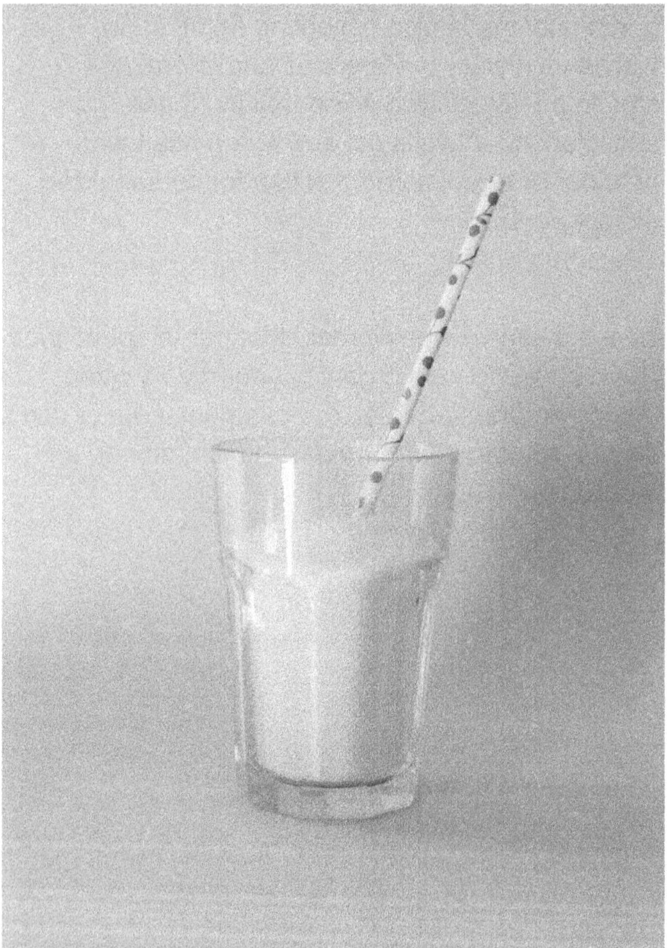

Weekly Meal Planner

```
---------------------------------------------------
Day:       | Monday       | Tuesday       | Wednesday
| Thursday      | Friday       | Saturday      | Sunday
|
---------------------------------------------------
Breakfast: |            |            |            |
|            |            |            |
---------------------------------------------------
Snack:     |            |            |            |
|            |            |            |
---------------------------------------------------
Lunch:     |            |            |            |
|            |            |            |
---------------------------------------------------
Snack:     |            |            |            |
|            |            |            |
---------------------------------------------------
Dinner:    |            |            |            |            |
|            |            |
---------------------------------------------------
Snack:     |            |            |            |
|            |            |            |
---------------------------------------------------
Notes:
```

Feel free to fill in the spaces with your meal choices, and use the "Notes" section to jot down any special considerations or reminders. Planning your meals in advance can help you make healthier choices, manage portion sizes, and maintain stable blood sugar levels while managing pre-diabetes.

www.ingramcontent.com/pod-product-compliance
Lightning Source LLC
Chambersburg PA
CBHW050017270826
50514CB00026B/347
9798866553037